ESSENTIAL

HERBAL
REMEDIES

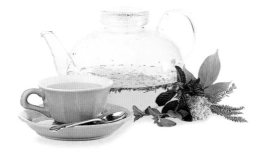

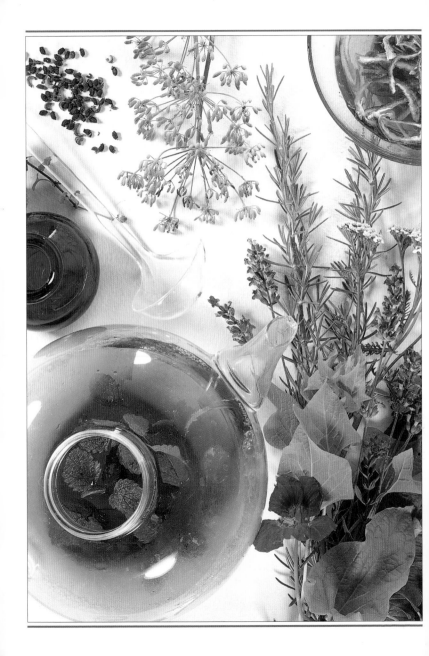

ESSENTIAL TIPS

HERBAL REMEDIES

Penelope Ody

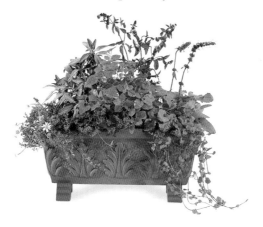

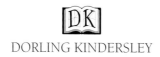

DORLING KINDERSLEY

DORLING KINDERSLEY
LONDON, NEW YORK, AUCKLAND, DELHI,
JOHANNESBURG, MUNICH, PARIS, SYDNEY

DK www.dk.com

Editor Bella Pringle
Art Editor Colin Walton
DTP Designer Robert Campbell
Senior Editor Peter Jones
Senior Art Editor Heather McCarry
Managing Editor Anna Kruger
Managing Art Editor Stephen Knowlden
Production Controller Louise Daly

First published in Great Britain in 2000 by
Dorling Kindersley Limited, 9 Henrietta Street, London WC2E 8PS

Copyright © 2000 Dorling Kindersley Limited, London
Text Copyright © 2000 Penelope Ody

All rights reserved. No part of this publication may be reproduced,
stored in a retrieval system, or transmitted in any form or by any means,
electronic, mechanical, photocopying, recording or otherwise, without
the prior written permission of the copyright owner.

A CIP catalogue record for this book is available from the British Library

ISBN 0-7513-2007-X

Text film output by Colourscan
Reproduced by Colourscan
Printed by Wing King Tong, Hong Kong

ESSENTIAL TIPS

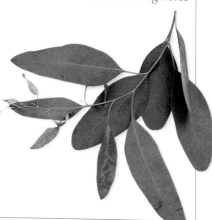

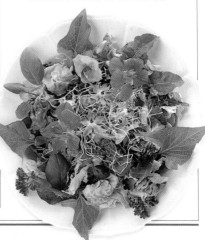

THE HEALING POWER OF HERBS

1 WHAT IS A HERB?

A herb may be broadly defined as any plant that is of some practical use, be it medicinal or culinary. Herbs include plants used in orthodox drugs, such as foxglove or opium poppy, as well as those that are familiar in the home, such as garlic or sage. The categorization of plants as herbs, vegetables, or weeds first occurred in the 17th century. Earlier cultures did not distinguish in the same way between foods and medicine.

FOXGLOVE REMEDY ▷
Foxglove was first identified as a heart remedy in 1768, and was the source of two major drugs. Many herbs have since proved valuable to the drugs industry.

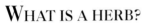
MEADOWSWEET ▽
This was the source of the first patent drug in the 1890s, aspirin. The herb is still used for fevers.

▽ ECHINACEA
Long used by the Native Americans, today the coneflower is valued as a natural antibiotic.

2 WHAT ARE HERBAL REMEDIES?

Since ancient times, herbs have played a vital role in medicine. While major illnesses have always been referred to specialist healers, self-limiting ailments were traditionally treated within the family, using herbal remedies passed down through generations. In many parts of the world, this is still the case; in the Western world, where there is increasing concern about the side-effects of modern orthodox drugs, interest in herbal medicine is growing.

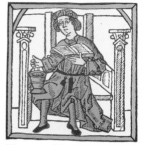

MEDIEVAL MEDICINE
In the Middle Ages, monks and apothecaries used herbal remedies to cure the sick.

3 HERBAL & CONVENTIONAL MEDICINE

Modern drugs may effect rapid apparent cures, but they do not solve the underlying cause of many problems, such as poor diet or lack of exercise. Herbal medicine is not just about curing illness when it occurs; it is also about prevention of illness, taking responsibility for our own well-being, and helping the body to heal itself.

USEFUL PLANT PARTS
The chemicals and thus the therapeutic properties of a herb are found in different parts of the plant. In lavender, it is the flowers and essential oil that are most important.

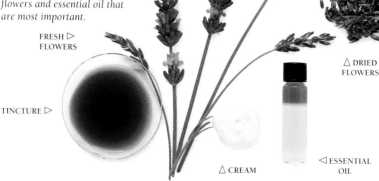

FRESH ▷ FLOWERS

TINCTURE ▷

△ DRIED FLOWERS

△ CREAM

◁ ESSENTIAL OIL

4 IS IT SAFE TO TREAT YOURSELF?

Herbalism has always been regarded as the "medicine of the people": simple remedies that can be used reliably at home for minor ills. Although most herbs are intrinsically quite safe, they should be treated with caution. Do not exceed the stated doses or continue with home remedies if conditions are worsening or persistent. If there is no improvement, or if there is any question of the accuracy of the diagnosis, do not delay in seeking professional help.

Standard adult doses must be reduced for babies, children, and the elderly (see Tip 42). If you have any concerns at all, it is wise to consult a professional practitioner.

5 WHEN TO AVOID HERBAL REMEDIES

Although herbal remedies are generally very safe, you should always observe these cautions:

▪ During pregnancy, some doses should be cut, and many herbs should be avoided entirely (*see Tip 89*). Avoid all medication in the first three months of pregnancy and take professional advice.

▪ If you suffer from certain disorders, you should avoid particular herbs. If you are epileptic, for example, avoid sage; if you have high blood pressure, avoid liquorice.

▪ Some herbs will interact with orthodox drugs. If on prescribed medication, consult a professional before attempting home remedies.

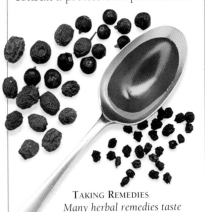

TAKING REMEDIES
Many herbal remedies taste bitter. Introduce them to babies and children early so they become accustomed to the taste.

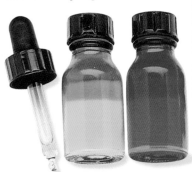

ESSENTIAL OILS
Do not take essential oils internally without professional medical supervision. Before taking them externally, dilute in a carrier oil. Always buy a reputable brand of commercially produced oils.

6 HERBS IN THE KITCHEN

Today's categorization of plants as herbs, vegetables, and fruits is fairly recent. To the 17th-century cook, cabbage, cucumber, and carrots were all "kitchen herbs".

The active constituents, such as alkaloids or saponins, present in herbs are also contained in other foods: fruit and vegetables can be therapeutic, or damaging in excess.

◁ CABBAGE
In folk medicine, cabbage was a standby for almost all the family ills.

GARLIC & ONIONS ▽ ▷
Raw onion soothes insect stings and garlic has long been known to lower blood cholesterol levels.

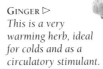

◁ CELERY
Eating fresh celery stalks can help to stimulate a mother's milk flow after birth.

GINGER ▷
This is a very warming herb, ideal for colds and as a circulatory stimulant.

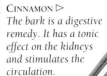

CHILLIES ▷
These are a potent stimulant for the whole body, and are antibacterial, ideal for colds and chills.

CINNAMON ▷
The bark is a digestive remedy. It has a tonic effect on the kidneys and stimulates the circulation.

◁ ORANGES
These relieve indigestion and nausea. Bergamot oil, from the peel of a dwarf orange tree, is used in aromatherapy.

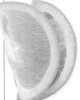

LEMONS ▷
The fruit is anti-inflammatory and anti-histaminic. Slices or juice can soothe sore skin.

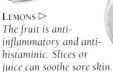

APPLES △
"An apple a day keeps the doctor away" – fresh apples are cleansing for the system.

7 HERBAL FIRST AID

Although we are more inclined to reach for patent antiseptics and pain-killers in a domestic emergency, herbs can provide effective alternatives to many over-the-counter pharmaceutical offerings. Herbal remedies can be bought ready-made in a variety of different forms, including creams, essential oils, and capsules. Raw ingredients found in most kitchen storecupboards, such as garlic, ginger, and herbal tea, also provide some useful first aid remedies.

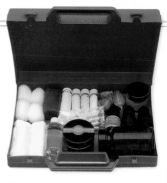

FIRST AID BOX
Keep herbal first aid remedies in a sealed box in a cool place out of the reach of children.

REMEDIES FOR THE KIT ▷
These are the most useful herbal remedies to keep in your kit at home. Most will last for a year or more without deterioration.

△ MARIGOLD CREAM

△ COMFREY OINTMENT

△ CHICKWEED CREAM

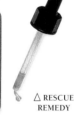
△ RESCUE REMEDY

ARNICA CREAM ▽

ARNICA 6X TABLETS ▷

EVENING PRIMROSE CAPSULES ▽

△ SLIPPERY ELM TABLETS

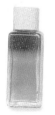
△ LAVENDER OIL

△ TEA TREE OIL

◁ DISTILLED WITCH HAZEL

△ ECHINACEA CAPSULES

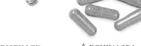

8 HERBS FOR HOLIDAYS

Holidays can be easily spoiled by minor ailments. Basic hygiene is essential in exotic locations. If you are prone to upsets, always peel fruit and do not eat any other raw foods; never drink tapwater. For upset stomachs and diarrhoea, eat papaya and drink strong black sugarless tea. Take a first aid kit stocked with the remedies shown.

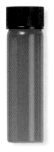

△ ST JOHN'S WORT & LAVENDER OIL

△ TEA TREE OIL

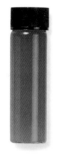

△ ST JOHN'S WORT & MARIGOLD TINCTURE

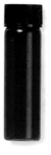

△ MEADOW-SWEET TINCTURE

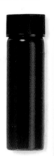

△ HONEYSUCKLE, BISTORT, & MARSHMALLOW TINCTURE

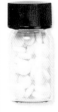

△ ARNICA 6x TABLETS

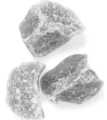

△ CRYSTALLIZED GINGER

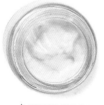

△ ARNICA CREAM

CHAMOMILE TEABAGS ▷

9 TRAVEL SICKNESS

Nausea and vomiting related to motion is especially common in childhood. Peppermint and ginger help to prevent vomiting. Take 1–2 x 200mg ginger capsules before travelling; alternatively, eat ginger biscuits, drink ginger ale, or chew crystallized ginger. For older children only, sucking sugar-free peppermint sweets also helps.

GROWING YOUR OWN HERBS

10 USEFUL HERBS TO GROW

Grow the following as the basis for a medicinal herb garden: chamomile (encourages sleep); fennel (aids digestion); hyssop (used in chest remedies); lemon balm (leaves make an antidepressant tea); pot marigold (a healing, astringent herb); purple sage (used in mouth-washes); rosemary (treats arthritis); St John's wort (treats burns); skullcap (a sedative for stress); and thyme (one of the best antiseptics).

USEFUL GARDEN HERBS
Many of these herbs not only have valuable medicinal and culinary properties, but they make good garden plants as well. Some may need to be protected with straw in winter.

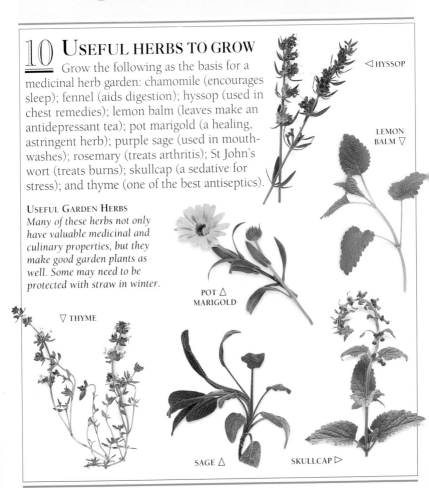

◁ HYSSOP

LEMON BALM ▽

POT △ MARIGOLD

▽ THYME

SAGE △

SKULLCAP ▷

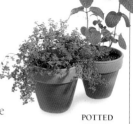

11 SOURCES OF SUPPLY

While it is satisfying to grow herbs from seeds or cuttings, this is not always practical. You can buy established plants from a good specialist nursery instead. Look for healthy, pest-free plants with a good root system (to check, slide the plant out of an upturned pot). Aim to buy in mid- to late spring before herbs become pot-bound.

POTTED HERBS

12 GROWING HERBS FROM SEED

Annual herbs are best grown from seed. Many perennial herbs can be grown from seed too; those that cannot may be grown from cuttings instead (see Tip 13).

- Annual and biennial herbs to grow from seed: angelica, anise, basil, borage, California poppy, coriander, corn salad, dill, mullein, nasturtium, parsley, pot marigold, and rocket.
- Perennial herbs to grow from seed: elecampane, fennel, feverfew, hyssop, lady's mantle, sage, St John's wort, self-heal, skullcap, and thyme.

POT MARIGOLD
Grow this annual from seed and harvest the flowers from early summer, often to early autumn.

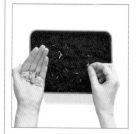

1 Sow annual seeds in spring where you wish them to grow. For perennials, fill a seedtray with compost that is well watered and sprinkle on the seeds.

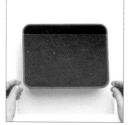

2 Cover large seeds with a thin layer of compost, then place a sheet of glass over the tray. Alternatively, put the tray in a plastic bag and store in a warm place.

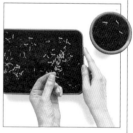

3 When the seedlings emerge, fill a pot with compost. Gently pick out some seedlings and insert them into tiny holes in the compost. Carefully firm the soil.

13 TAKING CUTTINGS

◁ SAGE

Woody perennial herbs can be propagated by cuttings rather than from seed. Cuttings can be selected from the side shoots of bushy herbs, such as sage or rosemary, when the shoots are semi-ripe (not quite woody) in late summer or early autumn, or from the new softwood (still fleshy) growth in spring and early summer. Softwood growth must develop fast for the cutting to survive; for this reason, semi-ripe cuttings are more likely to be successful.

▽ ROSEMARY

Some herbs, such as chives, lovage, and lemon balm, are best propagated by dividing the roots of existing plants to make two plants.

HERBS TO GROW FROM CUTTINGS ▷
As well as sage, rosemary, and lavender,
you can take semi-ripe cuttings of elder,
hyssop, lemon verbena, and thyme.

LAVENDER ▷

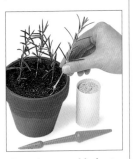

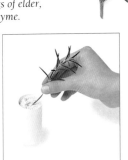

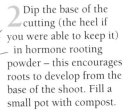

1 Select a suitable shoot (here, rosemary), and break or cut it off, keeping a heel of the main stem attached.

Heel at base

2 Dip the base of the cutting (the heel if you were able to keep it) in hormone rooting powder – this encourages roots to develop from the base of the shoot. Fill a small pot with compost.

3 Make several holes in the compost using a dibber (or the end of a pencil) and insert a cutting into each one. Water. After a few weeks, when roots appear, pot each cutting on.

14 PRUNING & CONTROLLING HERBS

Some herbs grow very rapidly and need vigorous pruning. Cutting plants regularly to dry for medicinal use keeps many under control. Be especially careful to control self-seeders, such as feverfew, lady's mantle, and lemon balm. Soapwort and mint have invasive root systems, so keep them firmly in check.

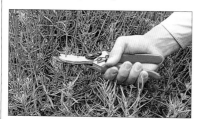

1 When pruning, or harvesting flowers or aerial parts for medicinal use, cut the plants back to 10–15cm (4–6in) high (or to the same length of new growth for woody herbs, like lavender).

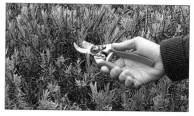

2 Early in spring, cut back the softwood shoots of woody perennial herbs by 2.5cm (1in). Make sure that some green growth remains: new shoots will not grow from old wood.

15 HERBS FOR A CLEAN ENVIRONMENT

Modern research has shown that many plants absorb polluting chemicals from the atmosphere and convert them to harmless substances. Growing plants in offices and homes can therefore help improve the environment for the people working and living there. Aloe vera absorbs many pollutants, while spider plants, azaleas, and weeping figs remove formaldehyde, found in building materials, cleaning agents, and cigarette smoke. Common ivy clears benzine emitted in some car exhaust fumes.

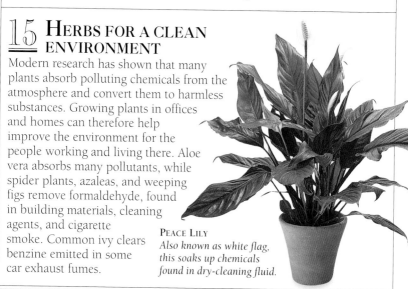

PEACE LILY
Also known as white flag, this soaks up chemicals found in dry-cleaning fluid.

17

16 HERB GARDEN IN A CONTAINER

Those with limited space may like to plant medicinal herbs in a windowbox. Herbs will grow happily for one or two seasons in containers, but a fresh planting each spring is preferable. Choose slow-growing varieties, and remember that herbs thrive in poor soil, so use a loam-based compost and ensure there is good drainage.

MEDICINAL WINDOWBOX
Plant taller herbs at the back, trailing plants near the edge at the front and sides, and small plants near the front. Variegated herbs make an attractive alternative.

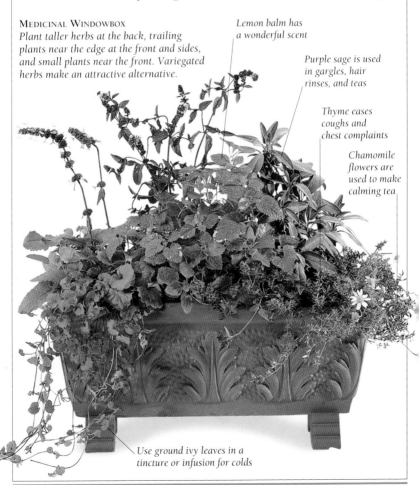

Lemon balm has a wonderful scent

Purple sage is used in gargles, hair rinses, and teas

Thyme eases coughs and chest complaints

Chamomile flowers are used to make calming tea

Use ground ivy leaves in a tincture or infusion for colds

GATHERING & PREPARING

17 BUYING DRIED HERBS

If you cannot grow the herbs you need, buy them dried from a reputable source instead.

- Always buy in small quantities to prevent lengthy storage.
- Do not buy from shops where herbs are stored in clear glass jars in direct sunlight, or where herbs look as though they have been on the shelves for a long time.
- Poorly harvested and stored herbs can become contaminated: check carefully for any sign.

DRIED HERBS
Good-quality dried herbs should show no sign of mould, mouse droppings, or insect infestations.

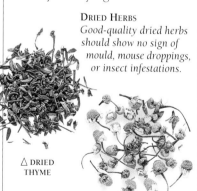

△ DRIED THYME

CHAMOMILE FLOWERS ▷

18 HANDLE WITH CARE!

Some healing plants are highly toxic. Eating deadly nightshade berries and hemlock can be fatal. Borage, chamomile, greater celandine, hops, primulas, rue, runner beans, and yarrow can cause rashes. Holly, laburnum, mistletoe, privet, spindle, sweet pea, and white bryony have toxic fruits. Do not swallow henbane.

MONKSHOOD
This plant is poisonous. Just touching it can cause numbness in the fingers.

19 WHEN TO GATHER FRESH HERBS

Seasonal growing patterns mean that it is often not possible to use fresh herbs all year round. Crops have to be harvested, dried, and stored for use when fresh plants are unavailable. When herbs are harvested can affect the composition of active chemicals considerably. They should be collected on a dry day, after the dew has dried, at the peak of their maturity to ensure the concentration of active ingredients is at its highest.

Most herbs are harvested in the summer, either before or during flowering. Seeds and most types of bark are collected in early autumn, and roots in early autumn or spring. Evergreen leaves, like rosemary, can be gathered throughout the year.

DANDELION
Gather dandelion leaves in early to midsummer, before the flowers appear.

SEASON	PARTS TO GATHER
Spring	**Roots** dandelion. **Aerial parts (while flowering)** lungwort, sweet violet. **Flowers** coltsfoot, cowslip, elder.
Early summer	**Aerial parts (while flowering)/leaves (before flowering)** agrimony, angelica, catmint, cleavers, dandelion, dill, fennel, feverfew, garlic, hyssop, lady's mantle, lemon balm, motherwort, parsley, peppermint, plantain, sage, stinging nettle, white horehound, yellow dock. **Bark (while flowering)** guelder rose. **Flowers/flowering tops** borage, chamomile, honeysuckle, linden, pot marigold, St John's wort.
Late summer	**Aerial parts (while flowering)** Californian poppy, heartsease, marjoram, marshmallow, meadowsweet, melilot, mugwort, shepherd's purse, skullcap, thyme, vervain, wild lettuce, wood betony, wormwood, yarrow. **Flowers** hops, lavender, mullein. **Leaves (after flowering)** borage, coltsfoot, cowslip, fenugreek, lungwort, sweet violet.
Autumn	**Roots/bulbs (when leaves have wilted)** angelica, black cohosh, burdock, comfrey, cowslip, elecampane, garlic, goldenseal, lovage, marshmallow, coneflower, soapwort, tormentil, valerian. **Seeds/fruit (when ripe)** bitter orange, celery, dill, elder, fennel, fenugreek, hawthorn, lovage.

20 DRYING FRESH HERBS

Herbs should always be dried as quickly as possible, in order to avoid valuable aromatic chemicals evaporating, and to limit the oxidization of important constituents. Dry them quickly, away from bright sunlight, and allowing plenty of air to circulate. Keep the temperature between 20–32°C (70–90°F). An airing cupboard with the door open, or a warm, dry garden shed, is ideal. The majority of herbs can be dried completely within 5–6 days, but seeds take longer. Do not use a microwave oven or dry them in garages (petrol fumes may contaminate the herbs).

21 DRYING FRESH FLOWERS

Generally, flowerheads are best gathered when the plant is in full bloom. Harvest them in the morning, after the dew has dried, and when they are fully open. Flowers are usually dried whole. Carefully cut each flowerhead off the stalk, remove any insects or grit from the surface of the petals, and place them on a tray lined with absorbent paper.

LAVENDER FLOWERS ▷
Small flowers, such as lavender, are dried using the same method as for seeds. Hang the stems upside down in a warm place, and collect the dried flowers in a paper bag.

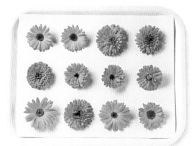

1 Place the flowerheads on a paper-lined tray. Leave them to dry in a warm place, such as an airing cupboard. Turn the flowers regularly.

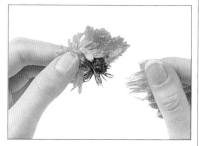

2 When the flowers are fully dry, store in a dark, airtight container. If using pot marigolds, remove the dried petals from the flower centre before storing.

22 SEEDS

It is best to collect seeds in the early autumn, when they are almost ripe, and before too many have been eaten by birds or dispersed by the wind. Harvest whole seedheads, leaving about 15–20cm (6–8in) of stalk. Tie the stalks in small bunches with string, and hang them upside down over a paper-lined tray. When the seeds are dry, they will fall off. An alternative method is to place a paper bag over the hanging seedheads and collect the seeds in the bag (*see Tip 21*).

23 BERRIES OR FRUIT

Early autumn is the best time to harvest berries or fruit, when they are just ripe, and before they have become too soft to dry successfully. Collect the berries and lay them on paper-lined trays, discarding any with signs of mould. Turn on the oven to the lowest setting. Place the trays in the oven with the door ajar for 3–4 hours, then transfer them to a warm, dry place, such as an airing cupboard. Turn the berries or fruit regularly to ensure even drying.

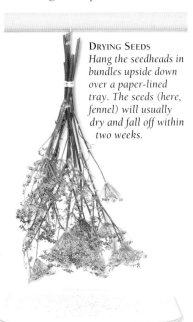

DRYING SEEDS
Hang the seedheads in bundles upside down over a paper-lined tray. The seeds (here, fennel) will usually dry and fall off within two weeks.

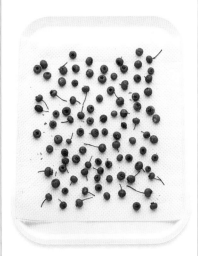

DRYING BERRIES
Spread the berries (here, hawthorn) on a paper-lined tray. Place the tray in a cooling oven, then transfer it to a warm place until the berries are dry.

24 LEAVES & AERIAL PARTS

Harvest leaves of deciduous herbs just before flowering. Evergreen herbs, such as rosemary, sage, and thyme, may be collected at any time of year, although avoid gathering large amounts when there is a risk of frost as it will damage the plant. You can harvest the large leaves of some herbs, such as burdock, individually; smaller leaves, such as those of lemon balm, are best dried on the stem. If you are using all of the aerial parts of a herb, harvest them in the early stages of flowering, so that you have a mixture of leaves, stems, flowers, and seedheads.

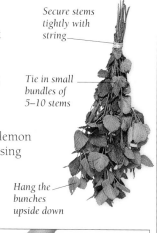

Secure stems tightly with string

Tie in small bundles of 5–10 stems

Hang the bunches upside down

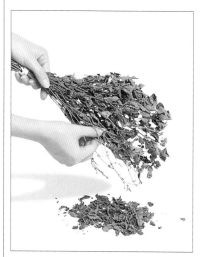

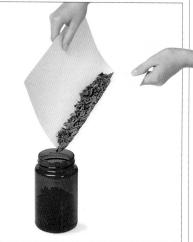

1 Hang the herb bunches (here, lemon balm) upside down in a warm room. After 5–6 days, when the leaves are brittle but not so dry that they turn to powder, rub them on to paper (discard larger pieces of stem). If using all aerial parts, crumble both leaves and stems.

2 When you have crumbled all the necessary plant parts, carefully pour or spoon the dried herbs from the piece of paper into an airtight, dark glass or ceramic storage jar. The container must be clean and dry, since herbs soon turn mouldy in damp conditions.

25 BULBS

To harvest bulbs, dig them up after flowering, as soon as the aerial parts have died down. It is important to collect garlic bulbs particularly quickly, since they have a tendency to sink down after the leaves have wilted, and so can quickly become buried and therefore difficult to find in the soil.

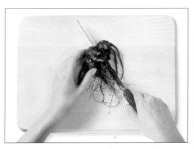

GARLIC BULB
Garlic is antibacterial and reduces cholesterol levels. It is a very valuable herb in old age.

Eat fresh garlic or 2–3 pearls daily

26 ROOTS

The majority of roots are best harvested in autumn, when the aerial parts have died down and before the ground becomes too hard to dig. Dandelions are an exception, and should be harvested in spring. After roots have dried completely, some tend to reabsorb moisture from the atmosphere, so it is essential to check them regularly and discard any that have become soft.

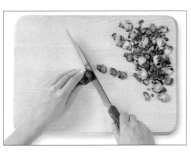

1 Select a plant with firm roots (here, marshmallow) and wash the roots thoroughly to remove soil and dirt. Dry well and place on a chopping board.

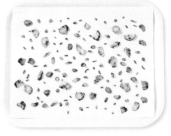

2 While they are still fresh, chop the large roots into small pieces using a kitchen knife. This will speed up the drying process. Line a tray with paper.

3 Lay the roots on the tray. Turn on the oven to the lowest setting. Put in the roots, leaving the door ajar, for 2–3 hours. Move to a warm place until dry.

27 PLANT SAP & GEL

You can collect sap from a number of plants. To collect sap from a tree, make a deep incision with a knife, or drill a hole into the bark, and collect the sap with a cup or bucket. Try to collect the sap in the autumn, in order to minimize damage to the tree. To collect sap from latex plants, such as wild lettuce and greater celandine, simply squeeze the plant over a bowl. Since some saps tend to be corrosive, it is advisable to wear a pair of protective gloves.

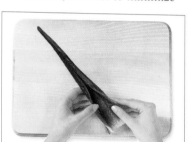

1 Gel from the aloe vera plant is very useful in first aid, and can also be used to make creams. To collect the gel from aloe, carefully slice along the centre of a leaf with a sharp knife, then peel back the edges.

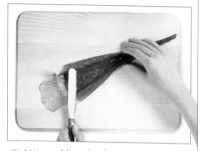

2 Using a blunt knife, or the blunt edge of a knife, scrape the gel from the leaf on to a clean surface. The thick gel, which is ideal for soothing minor burns, scalds, or sunburn, may then be applied directly to the affected area.

28 STORING HERBS

Most dried herbs will keep for up to a year, provided they are stored correctly. They require airtight, dry containers in cool conditions, away from direct sunlight. Dark glass or ceramic containers are best, but if you have clear glass jars, then make sure that you keep them in a dark cupboard. Inspect herbs often for signs of mould or insect infestation: eggs and chrysalises are common. Label containers with details of the variety, source, and date.

Tight-fitting cork stopper prolongs life of herbs

DARK GLASS BOTTLE

Dark glass keeps out bright light

MAKING & USING THE REMEDIES

29 EQUIPMENT

The equipment needed for making remedies is found in most kitchens. Use enamel, glass, stainless steel, cast iron, or pottery utensils. Never use aluminium pans or store herbal remedies in plastic containers for long periods.

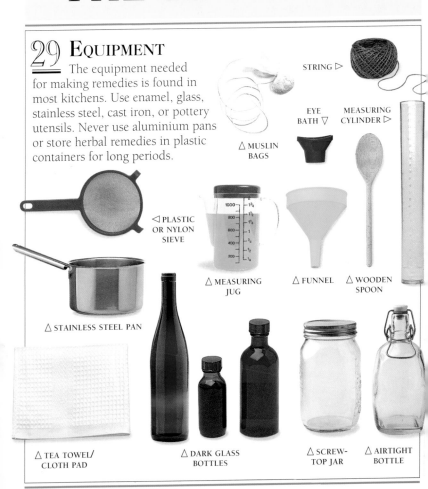

STRING ▷

EYE BATH ▽

MEASURING CYLINDER ▷

△ MUSLIN BAGS

◁ PLASTIC OR NYLON SIEVE

△ MEASURING JUG

△ FUNNEL

△ WOODEN SPOON

△ STAINLESS STEEL PAN

△ TEA TOWEL/ CLOTH PAD

△ DARK GLASS BOTTLES

△ SCREW-TOP JAR

△ AIRTIGHT BOTTLE

30 STERILIZING THE EQUIPMENT

All equipment must be kept clean, but storage jars should be sterilized before use, otherwise many herbal medicines – especially creams and syrups – will soon go mouldy. To sterilize glass containers, wash them thoroughly in freshly boiled water and place in a hot oven (at least 160°C/325°F/gas mark 3) for 1 hour. Handle with care when removing. Alternatively, use the preparations sold for baby's bottles or home wine-making. Before use, soak all storage bottles, jars, and lids for at least 30 minutes (or as specified on the label), then rinse with freshly boiled water and dry in a hot oven.

31 DIFFERENT TYPES OF REMEDY

Herbal remedies come in many forms. They may be taken orally (infusions, decoctions, syrups, juices, tinctures, tonics, capsules, gargles); internally (suppositories, pessaries); or used on the skin (compresses, poultices, ointments, lotions, creams, massage oils, in bath water).

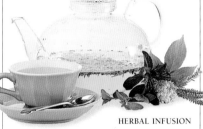

HERBAL INFUSION

32 DEFINING THE REMEDY

Remedies work in different ways on different parts of the body, and there are specific terms to describe these effects. The following are commonly used: a *bitter* stimulates secretion of digestive juices and encourages appetite; a *tonic* restores and nourishes the entire body; a *carminative* relieves flatulence, digestive colic, and gastric discomfort; and a *demulcent* softens and soothes damaged or inflamed surfaces, such as the gastric mucous membranes. Comfrey, for example, is a good demulcent.

MARSHMALLOW
This demulcent calms inflammation in the digestive tract and urinary system.

33 INFUSIONS

Infusions are taken as remedies for particular ailments, or can simply be enjoyed for their relaxing or revitalizing effects. They may be made from a single herb, or from a combination, and may be drunk hot or cold. Generally, take a teacup or wineglass dose 3 times daily, less for children and the elderly.

LEMON BALM
A good antidepressant and digestive herb, lemon balm makes a delicious infusion.

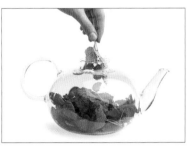

1 Warm a teapot with hot water. Add 25g dried herbs, or 75g fresh herbs (here, lemon balm). Use the leaves, flowers, and most aerial parts.

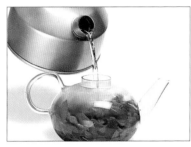

2 Pour over 500ml hot water that is just off the boil. Cover the teapot with the lid and leave the herbs to infuse in the water for 10 minutes.

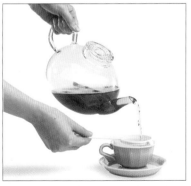

3 Strain the infusion through a nylon or plastic tea strainer. There should be enough for 3 doses in the pot.

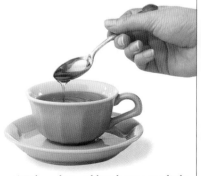

4 Take a dose, adding honey or a little unrefined sugar to taste. Strain the rest into a jug, cover, and store in a cool place or refrigerator for up to 48 hours.

34 DECOCTIONS

Some plant materials require more vigorous extraction than is possible with an infusion. The decoction method is ideal for tough parts such as barks, berries, or roots. Use herbs singly or in combination. The dosage is as for infusions.

LIQUORICE ROOT
A decoction made with dried liquorice root is an energy tonic, particularly for the digestive system. It is also used for coughs and ulcers.

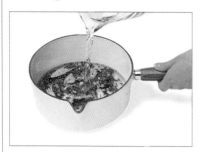

1 Place 60g fresh herbs or 30g dried herbs (here, liquorice root, *Gao Ben*, and devil's claw) in a pan. Add 750ml cold water.

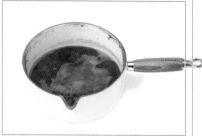

2 Place the pan on the heat and bring to the boil. Simmer gently for 20–40 minutes, until the volume has reduced by about one-third.

3 ◁ Take the decoction off the heat and strain through a nylon or plastic sieve into a heatproof jug. Taste, and add honey or unrefined sugar to sweeten if necessary. Alternatively, you may prefer to add a little lemon juice.

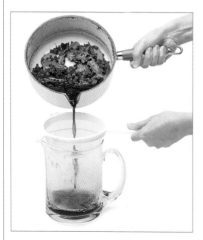

4 ▷ Pour the decoction into a covered jug, and store in a cool place or refrigerator for up to 48 hours. It may be drunk either cold or hot (repeat doses may be reheated).

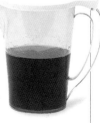

35 SYRUPS

Unrefined sugar or honey may be added to an infusion or decoction to make a syrup. Syrups disguise the flavour of some herbs and preserve the active ingredients.

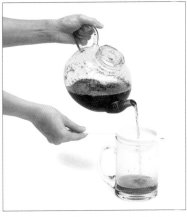

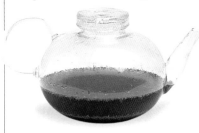

1 Make a 500ml standard infusion or decoction combining your chosen herbs (*see Tips 33 and 34*).

2 Using a small nylon or plastic sieve, strain the infusion (here, hyssop) or decoction into a jug, then pour into a clean saucepan.

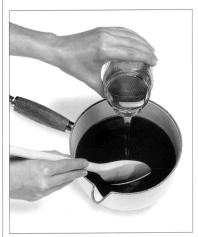

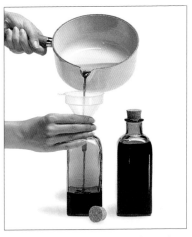

3 Add 500g runny honey or unrefined sugar and stir constantly until dissolved. Simmer gently until the mixture is syrupy, then allow to cool.

4 Pour the mixture into bottles and seal with a cork stopper. Avoid screw-top bottles, since syrups can ferment and the bottle could explode.

36 EYEBATHS

Simple to make and use, eyebaths are very soothing for many eye complaints. Use either weak infusions or decoctions, or add 2 drops of tincture to an eyebath filled with freshly boiled water. It is vital to sterilize the eyebath in between bathing each eye (*see Tip 30*).

◁ **MARIGOLD**
Astringent and antiseptic, pot marigold is an excellent remedy for inflammations, such as styes, as well as for local skin infections.

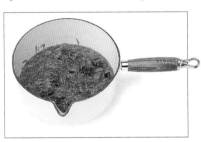

1 Make an infusion or decoction of your chosen herb (*see Tips 33 and 34*). Simmer for 10–15 minutes.

2 ▷ Strain the mixture thoroughly through a fine nylon or plastic sieve. Ensure there are no particles of herb remaining that might irritate the eye.

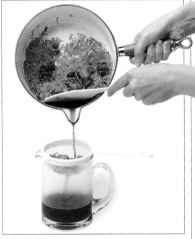

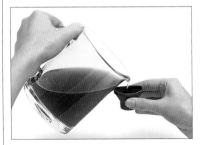

3 Leave the mixture to cool to a lukewarm temperature, and then fill a sterilized eyebath with the mixture.

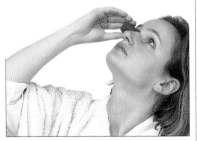

4 Place the eyebath over the eye, and tilt your head back so that the eye is thoroughly wetted. Blink several times.

37 TINCTURES

The advantage of tinctures is that the alcohol acts as a preservative, enabling the tincture to keep for 2 years. Vodka is ideal, but other spirits are also suitable, provided they are not toxic (never use methylated spirits).

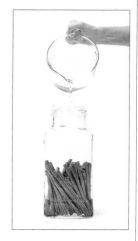

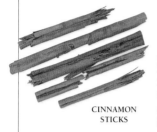

CINNAMON STICKS

1 ▷ Place 600g of fresh or 200g of dried herbs (here, cinnamon) in a jar. Add 650ml of vodka and 350ml water to make a 25% alcohol mixture. Seal the jar and store in a cool place for 2 weeks. Shake occasionally.

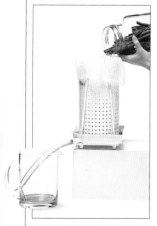

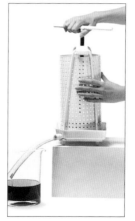

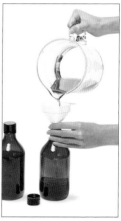

2 Place a muslin bag inside a wine press, wrapping the bag edges around the sides of the press to prevent it from slipping. Pour the alcohol, water, and herb mixture through the bag.

3 Holding the wine press firm with one hand, squeeze the mixture through the press into a jug. The residue of the mixture can be added to the garden compost heap.

4 Pour the strained liquid into sterilized, dark glass bottles, using a funnel. Take 5ml 3 times a day, diluted in a little warm water. A little honey or fruit juice can improve the flavour.

38 MASSAGE OILS

Massage is one of the most effective antidotes to stress, greatly enhancing our sense of well-being. Massage oils are easy to make from a few drops of essential oil diluted in a carrier oil – sweet almond or wheatgerm is best, but sunflower, vegetable, or infused oils may also be used. Essential oils do not last long once diluted, so make up small batches as and when you need them. Use no more than a 10% concentration of essential oils, 5% for children or the elderly or those with sensitive skins.

CAUTIONS
• *Do not massage anyone suffering from an infection, epilepsy, acute back pain, a contagious disease, or an inflammatory condition such as thrombosis.*
• *Pregnant women should seek professional advice before using essential oils.*

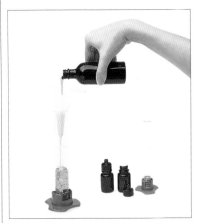

1 Measure out 45ml carrier oil (here, wheatgerm oil) into a large measuring cylinder and 5ml essential oils (here, lavender and thyme) into a small cylinder, using a funnel.

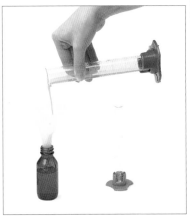

2 Carefully pour the carrier oil and the essential oil into a 50ml sterilized, dark glass bottle, again using the funnel. Replace the lid: it is essential that the bottle is airtight.

3 Shake the bottle to mix and then store in a cool place. To apply, pour about 2–5ml on to the hands (not directly on to the body) and rub gently.

Tight-fitting screw-top lid

39 COLD INFUSIONS OF OILS

Cold infused oils are used in massage oils or as the basis of creams or ointments. This method is suitable for flowers, such as melilot, pot marigold, or St John's wort. The flowers and oil are placed together in a jar and left to stand for 2–3 weeks to infuse; the once-infused oil is then used again with fresh herb to extract as much of the active ingredient as possible.

ST JOHN'S WORT

SUITABLE HERBS TO USE
• Melilot (dried herb): varicose eczema.
• Pot marigold (fresh or dried petals): grazes; dry eczema; fungal infections, such as thrush and athlete's foot.
• St John's wort (fresh flowering tops): sunburn; minor scalds and burns; grazes; inflamed joints.

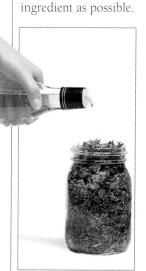

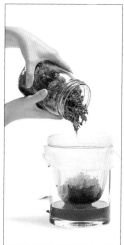

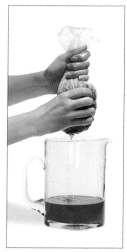

1 Pack a large jar tightly with the herb (here, St John's wort) and cover completely with cold-pressed safflower or walnut oil. Put the lid on and leave in a greenhouse or on a sunny windowsill for 2–3 weeks.

2 Remove the lid and pour or spoon the herb and oil mixture into a jelly bag fitted tightly with string or an elastic band to the rim of a jug. Alternatively, use a muslin bag and a wine press (see facing page).

3 Squeeze the oil through the bag. Repeat steps 1 and 2 with a new herb and the once-infused oil. After a few weeks, strain again and store in airtight, sterilized, dark glass bottles for up to a year.

40 Hot Infusions of Oils

Like cold infused oils, hot infused oils are used as the basis of creams, ointments, or massage oils. The hot infusion method is suitable for leafy herbs, such as chickweed, stinging nettle, and rosemary. Hot infusions will last for up to a year if stored in a cool, dark place.

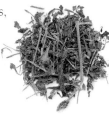

CHICKWEED
This eases burns, scalds, eczema, and insect stings.

SUITABLE HERBS TO USE
• *Bladderwrack: arthritic pain.*
• *Chickweed: irritant eczema; burns; scalds.*
• *Cleavers: psoriasis.*
• *Comfrey: bruises; sprains; osteoarthritis.*
• *Stinging nettle: allergic skin rashes; eczema.*
• *Rosemary: aches and pains.*

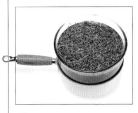

1 △ Place 500ml sunflower oil and 250g dried herb aerial parts and leaves (here, chickweed) in a glass bowl over a pan of simmering water, or in a double boiler. Heat gently for about 3 hours.

2 ▷ Strain the oil and dried herb mixture through a muslin bag fitted to a wine press into a jug. An alternative method is to strain it through a jelly bag attached to the rim of a jug (see facing page).

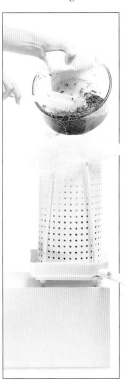

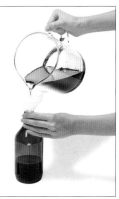

3 △ Pour the oil into sterilized, airtight, dark glass bottles. Store in a cool, dark place for up to a year.

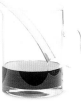

41 COMPRESSES

A compress is simply a cloth soaked in a bowl of hot or cold herbal extract, either an infusion, a decoction, or a tincture diluted with hot or cold water. Compresses help to ease the strain of painful joints and muscles, and also help soothe skin rashes and irritations.

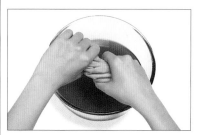

1 Soak a clean tea towel or muslin in a 500ml standard infusion (here, arnica) or decoction, or 50ml tincture in 500ml hot or cold water. Squeeze out the excess liquid.

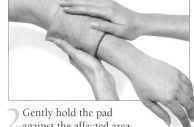

2 Gently hold the pad against the affected area. When it cools or dries, repeat the process using hot mixture. You can apply the compress as often as required.

42 TREATMENT & DOSAGE

The recipes and remedies featured in this book are safe, but exceeding the recommended dose can be harmful. All the dosages given are for adults, and so need to be reduced in some cases. Follow the guidelines set out below:

• For children under 2 years, give one-fifth of the adult dose, increasing gradually (depending on the size of the child) to reach a quarter at age 3 or 4, a third at 6 or 7, a half at 8 or 9, and increasing to the full adult dose at puberty.

• The elderly may require lower doses than younger adults owing to

MEASURING SPOONS
A set of spoons is ideal for measuring out smaller quantities of herbs and liquids.

their usually slower metabolism. Reduce doses by half for the very elderly or those who are particularly frail.

• Pregnant women should avoid taking any medication in the first 3 months of pregnancy, and must consult a professional practitioner before taking any home remedies, since certain herbs can be harmful in pregnancy (*see Tip 89*).

TONIC HERBS

43 BODY, MIND, & SPIRIT

Holistic medicine focuses on the needs of the body, mind, and spirit, and this is particularly true of any nervous disorder. Nervous complaints may be physical, emotional, or spiritual. Herbs can operate on all three levels to cure numerous disorders such as anxiety, panic attacks, and tension.

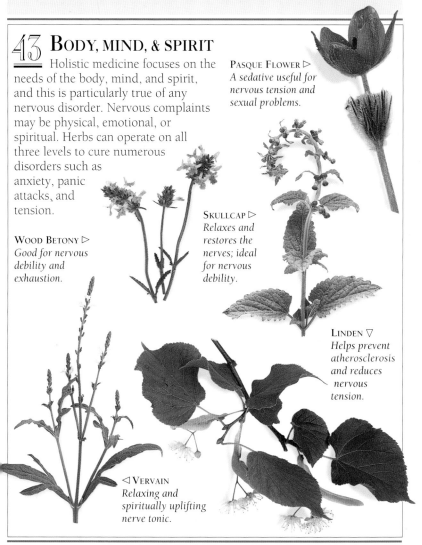

PASQUE FLOWER ▷
A sedative useful for nervous tension and sexual problems.

WOOD BETONY ▷
Good for nervous debility and exhaustion.

SKULLCAP ▷
Relaxes and restores the nerves; ideal for nervous debility.

LINDEN ▽
Helps prevent atherosclerosis and reduces nervous tension.

◁ **VERVAIN**
Relaxing and spiritually uplifting nerve tonic.

44 SALAD HERBS

Salad herbs are greatly valued for their highly beneficial properties. They have a wide range of therapeutic actions: fennel eases indigestion, chicory is a good bile stimulant and laxative, and watercress is a rich source of minerals and vitamins. Raw sliced vegetables, such as cabbage which helps treat arthritis and threadworms, are also excellent for the digestion.

SALAD ROCKET ▷
This salad herb adds a distinctive peppery flavour to salads, and is a good source of vitamin C. It is also mildly diuretic.

◁ DANDELION
Rich in potassium, dandelion leaves are an effective diuretic, and also a good liver and digestive tonic.

◁ WATERCRESS
Commonly used as garnish, watercress is rich in minerals and vitamin C; as a result, it is an excellent tonic for anaemia.

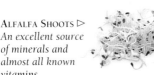

ALFALFA SHOOTS ▷
An excellent source of minerals and almost all known vitamins.

CORIANDER ▷
A popular Indian remedy for digestive upsets and urinary tract infections.

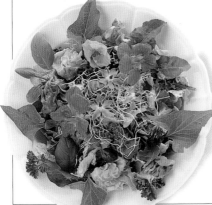

45 TONIC SALAD

This mixture contains herbs that provide plenty of vitamins and minerals, and that also stimulate the liver and adrenal glands.

- Combine some lettuce leaves and a few alfalfa sprouts. Add the following leaves, roughly shredded: basil, dandelion, good King Henry, parsley.
- Toss in an olive oil and lemon juice dressing and decorate with nasturtium and borage flowers.

46 SALAD FOR DIGESTION

A delicious salad that combines carminative herbs, used for easing digestion and gastric discomfort, with gentle bile stimulants that give a mild laxative effect to help regulate the digestive system.

- Finely slice a fennel bulb and combine it in a bowl with washed chicory leaves. Add just a small handful of lemon balm leaves and 1–2 shredded alecost leaves.
- Toss the salad in a dressing made from olive oil and lemon juice and decorate the salad with a sprinkling of sesame seeds or rocket flowers.

Note: Do not confuse alecost leaves with those of the camphor plant, which are similar in appearance.

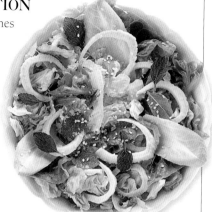

HEALTHY ACCOMPANIMENT
A large bowl of green salad acts as an excellent spring-clean for those with sluggish digestions.

47 TEAS TO NOURISH & RESTORE

Also known as herbal infusions, herbal teas are taken to treat specific ailments, as well as making a delicious, healthy, caffeine-free alternative to tea or coffee. You can dry fresh herbs at home, and make up your own concoctions. Alternatively, ready-made teabags are available in a wide range of flavours from healthfood shops and supermarkets. However, commercial blends tend to rely on berries and fruit peel for taste, and they can also contain large amounts of sugar. In some conditions, such as candidiasis, these are best avoided. When making teas or infusions, the water must be just off the boil, since vigorously boiling water disperses valuable volatile oils in the steam. Try to keep a separate teapot for making herbal infusions.

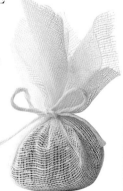

HOMEMADE BAGS
Make your own tea bags by wrapping dried herbs in a piece of muslin.

48 MORNING TEA
Peppermint & hibiscus tea

Ingredients
25g dried
peppermint leaves
50g dried hibiscus flowers
50g dried & crushed
strawberry leaves
25g dried & crushed
raspberry leaves
25g dried marigold petals
25g dried
chamomile flowers
25g dried cornflowers
water

This combination contains stimulating and digestive herbs to provide a refreshing and reviving start to the day.

1 Mix and store the herbs in a dark glass or ceramic jar. Place 1–2 tsp in a tisane cup or small teapot.

2 Add a cup of freshly boiled water and infuse for 5–10 minutes. Strain. Drink first thing in the morning for a good start.

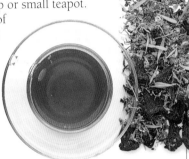

49 UPLIFTING TEA
Vervain & linden flower tea

Ingredients
25g dried
chamomile flowers
50g dried vervain
50g dried peppermint
leaves
50g dried & crushed
linden flowers
25g dried lavender flowers
25g dried lemon
balm leaves
water

A restoring brew to improve happiness and well-being, with herbs traditionally believed to lift the spirits. Peppermint teas, which help indigestion and headcolds, and chamomile teas, which relax and soothe, are widely available commercially.

1 Mix the herbs and store in a dark jar. Place 1–2 tsp in a tisane cup or small teapot.

2 Add a cup of freshly boiled water and infuse for 5–10 minutes. Strain.

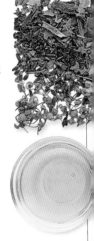

50 RELAXING MIXTURE
Lemon balm & chamomile tea

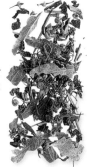

Ingredients
*50g dried lemon
balm leaves
50g dried
chamomile leaves
50g dried & crushed
linden flowers
water*

Try this calming mixture of sedating herbs to help unwind after a hard day's work. Lemon balm is a good digestive and antidepressant, chamomile soothes and relaxes, and linden is a useful sedative for nervous tension and anxiety, as well as a good remedy for high blood pressure associated with stress and fevers.

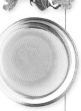

1 Mix and store the herbs in a dark glass or ceramic jar. Place 1–2 tsp in a tisane cup or small teapot.
2 Add a cup of freshly boiled water and infuse for 5–10 minutes. Strain and drink to help you relax.

51 NIGHTCAP TEA
Poppy & wild lettuce tea

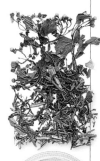

Ingredients
*25g dried
Californian poppies
50g dried wild
lettuce leaves
25g dried
hawthorn flowers
25g dried melilot
water*

A hot infusion of relaxing herbs can be just the thing to guarantee a good night's sleep. This mixture is adapted from a recipe of the great French herbalist, Maurice Mességué.
1 Combine and store the herbs in a dark glass or ceramic jar. Place 1–2 tsp in a tisane cup or small teapot.

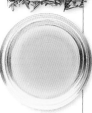

2 Add a cup of freshly boiled water and infuse for 5–10 minutes. Strain. Drink hot before going to bed.

MINOR AILMENTS

52 SORE THROAT & LARYNGITIS
Sage & rosemary gargle

Ingredients
15g dried or 45g fresh
red sage leaves
10g dried or 20g fresh
rosemary leaves
5g dried lady's
mantle leaves
500ml water

DOSAGE
While symptoms persist,
gargle with a wineglass
dose every 2–3 hours.
Swallow the tea after
gargling.

One of the best combinations for sore throats
and laryngitis is a sage and rosemary gargle.
Both rosemary and sage are aromatic, antiseptic,
and rich in potent healing oils. Additional
astringents, such as lady's mantle, can also help
reduce inflammation.

1 Mix the herbs together in a teapot or jug and
add freshly boiled water.

2 Infuse for 10 minutes, strain, and allow the
mixture to cool. Cover and store in a cool place.

Other treatments
■ Add 1 tsp of echinacea tincture (see Tip 37) to
each gargle or take alone to combat infections.
■ Take 2–3 garlic pearls daily to support the
immune system.
■ Mix 2 drops each of sandalwood,
frankincense, and lavender essential oils with
1 tsp sweet almond oil and massage the mixture
around the throat.

CAUTIONS FOR COUGHS
• Persistent or recurrent coughs, at any
age, can be a sign of more serious health
problems. Seek professional help if the
cough lasts for more than a week or so,
if there is chest pain, or if there is no
obviously associated cold or infection.
• If the phlegm from a cough is streaked
with blood, or the infection is slow
to clear, consult your doctor.

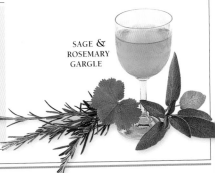

SAGE &
ROSEMARY
GARGLE

53 COMMON COLD
Boneset & elderflower tea

Ingredients
10g dried boneset
10g dried elderflower
5g dried yarrow
5g dried peppermint
500ml water
DOSAGE
Take a wineglass dose
every 3–4 hours, as long
as symptoms persist.

Boneset was used in North America for bone-shaking fevers. Elderflower combats catarrh.
1 Mix the herbs and place in a teapot and pour on the freshly boiled water.
2 Infuse for 10 minutes and strain into a jug. Cover and store in a cool place.

Other treatment
▪ If you feel cold and shivery, drink a warm decoction of ginger and other spicy herbs (*see Tip 34*).

ELDERFLOWER

54 HAYFEVER & ALLERGIC RHINITIS
Elderflower & dandelion tincture

Ingredients
25ml elderflower tincture
20ml dandelion root tincture
20ml vervain tincture
15ml Siberian ginseng tincture
15ml white horehound tincture
5ml liquorice tincture
DOSAGE
Take 5ml in 100ml warm water 3 times a day before meals.

This tincture, containing elderflower to strengthen the mucous membranes and dandelion to cleanse the liver, will help the system cope with future allergens and so reduce symptoms. For hayfever, take it for up to 4 weeks in early spring, before the pollen arrives.
1 To make the individual tinctures, see Tip 37.
2 Mix the tinctures together in a sterilized, dark glass bottle.

Other treatment
▪ To relieve hayfever, bathe eyes with a marigold and eyebright eye-bath (*see Tip 63*).

ELDERFLOWER & DANDELION TINCTURE

55 DIARRHOEA
Tormentil & marshmallow decoction

MARSHMALLOW
◁ ROOT

△ TORMENTIL
ROOT

Ingredients
1 tbsp arrowroot
15g dried
tormentil root
10g dried
marshmallow root
5g dried
cinnamon bark
750ml water

DOSAGE

Take a teacup dose 3
times a day until
symptoms subside.

This mixture of herbs and
arrowroot is soothing and
nutritious. Tormentil root is rich
in tannins and highly astringent,
helping to reduce inflammation,
while marshmallow is soothing.

1 Blend the arrowroot with 1 tbsp
of cold water to form a paste in a bowl or jug.
2 Simmer the herbs in the water for 10–15
minutes. Strain, return the liquid to the pan,
and bring to the boil.
3 Pour the boiling decoction over the blended
arrowroot, stirring well. Store in a cool place.

56 CONSTIPATION
Liquorice & dandelion decoction

Ingredients
10g dried dandelion root
5g dried yellow dock root
5g dried liquorice root
5g dried anise seeds
750ml water

DOSAGE

Take a wineglass dose
3 times a day.

Constipation often suggests a sluggish
digestion, which can be improved by
bitter herbs that stimulate the liver
and encourage production of digestive
enzymes. Dandelion is a good liver
tonic; yellow dock is a gentle laxative.
1 Put the herbs and water in a pan.
2 Bring to the boil and simmer gently
for 10 minutes, or until
reduced by about one-third.
Strain into a jug. Cover and
store in a cool place.

Other treatment
▪ Add 1 tsp of ispaghula
seeds to a cup of boiling
water. Infuse for 10
minutes, stir, then drink.

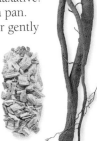

LIQUORICE △ ▷
ROOTS

57 INDIGESTION & HEARTBURN
Fennel & lemon balm tea

Ingredients
10g dried fennel seeds
*15g dried or 45g fresh
lemon balm leaves*
*2–3g dried cinnamon bark
or a pinch of powdered
cinnamon*
500ml water

DOSAGE
Take a wineglass dose
after meals as required.

Both fennel and lemon balm are very calming for the stomach, while lemon balm also helps relax the nerves if stress or anxiety is contributing to the problem.

1 Place the mixture of seeds, leaves, and bark in a teapot. Add freshly boiled water.

2 Leave the herbs to infuse for 10 minutes. Strain the surplus into a covered jug and store in a cool place.

Other treatments
- Take carminative teas regularly, such as chamomile, peppermint, fennel, or lemon balm.
- Slippery elm capsules can often soothe the effects of heartburn.

**FENNEL &
LEMON BALM TEA**

58 HAEMORRHOIDS
Pilewort ointment

Ingredients
75g dried pilewort leaves
500ml sunflower oil
25g beeswax
25g anhydrous lanolin

DOSAGE
Rub the ointment on the
piles several times a day.

Pilewort is a very astringent plant, and can be extremely helpful for relieving haemorrhoids.

1 Heat the pilewort and the oil in a double boiler, or over a waterbath, for 3 hours to make an infused oil, and strain the mixture through a jelly bag (*see Tip 39*).

2 Meanwhile, melt the beeswax and anhydrous lanolin in a separate saucepan.

3 Add 100ml of the warm infused oil to the melted wax mixture in the pan. Stir well and pour the ointment into sterilized jars before it starts to set. Rub into the affected areas.

59 ANXIETY & TENSION
Skullcap & passionflower mixture

Ingredients
50ml skullcap tincture
25ml passionflower tincture
15ml lemon balm tincture
10ml pasque flower tincture
DOSAGE
Take 5ml in a little warm water when feeling anxious or tense. Repeat up to 5 times a day.

Soothing herbal nervines encourage relaxation and reduce tensions. Skullcap is a restorative and relaxant, while passionflower has an effective sedative action.
1 Make the individual tinctures (*see Tip 37*).
2 Combine the tinctures in a sterilized, dark glass bottle. Shake the bottle well to mix thoroughly.

SKULLCAP

Other treatment
■ To prevent panic attacks, massage 5 drops of rose or neroli oil diluted in 1 tsp of sweet almond oil into the temples.

60 INSOMNIA
Poppy & passionflower tea

Ingredients
20g dried Californian poppy
15g dried passionflower
10g dried wood betony
5g dried lavender flowers
water
DOSAGE
Drink a cup about 30 minutes before you go to bed.

Californian poppies are also known as "nightcap" and were used as a sedative by Native Americans. This is a gentle, soothing remedy that is safe, even for children.
1 Mix the herbs and store in a dry, airtight container.
2 Put 2 tsp of the mixture in a tisane cup and add freshly boiled water. Infuse for 5–10 minutes. Strain and drink before bed.

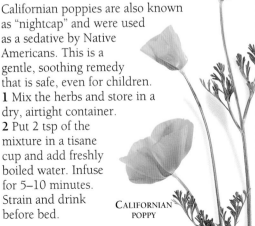

CALIFORNIAN POPPY

61 BACKACHE & SCIATICA
Lavender & thyme rub

Ingredients
10 drops lavender oil
10 drops thyme oil
5 drops juniper oil
10 drops eucalyptus oil
5 drops pine oil
18ml infused St John's wort oil
DOSAGE
Use 1 tsp oil and repeat at least twice a day.

HERBAL REMEDY
These oils relax tense muscles and relieve pain caused by backache.

Lavender oil is a mild analgesic and can help many types of backache, while thyme is an antispasmodic that relaxes over-tense muscles. Combined with warming oils, they can soothe aches and pains.

1 Select good-quality oils. To make the infused St John's wort oil, see Tip 39.

2 Combine the oils in a 20ml sterilized, airtight, dark glass bottle and shake thoroughly. Store for up to 3 months. To use, pour the oil on to one palm and rub your hands together before massaging very gently into the painful areas.

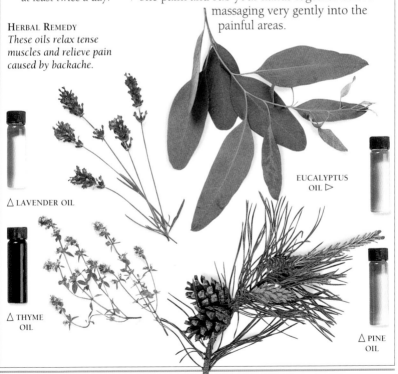

△ LAVENDER OIL

EUCALYPTUS OIL ▷

△ THYME OIL

△ PINE OIL

62 EYE STRAIN
Ju Hua & wood betony tea

Ingredients
25g Ju Hua (*dried,
prepared Chinese
chrysanthemum flowers*)
20g dried wood betony
10g dried gotu kola
5g dried peppermint
water

DOSAGE
Drink a cup whenever
your eyes feel tired.

In Chinese medicine, the
eyes are associated with
the liver. Herbs such as *Ju
Hua* and wood betony,
which work on the liver,
can also help the eyes.
1 Mix the herbs and store
in a dark, airtight bottle.
2 Put 2–3 tsp of the mix in
a tisane cup or small
teapot. Add a cup of freshly
boiled water and infuse for
10 minutes. Strain.

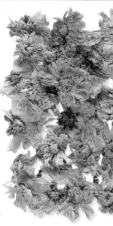

CHRYSANTHEMUM
FLOWERS

63 CONJUNCTIVITIS
Eyebright & marigold eyebath

Ingredients
15g dried eyebright
10g dried pot
marigold petals
500ml water

DOSAGE
Pour a little into an
eyebath. In acute cases,
repeat often.

CAUTION
*If the infection does not
clear in a day or so, or if
there is decreased vision
or pain, consult a doctor.*

Eyebright, as its name suggests, is a herb
traditionally used to treat eye infections. Make
up a fresh mixture each day; thorough
sterilization of equipment is vital (*see Tip 30*).

EYEBRIGHT

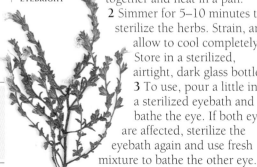

1 Mix the herbs and water
together and heat in a pan.
2 Simmer for 5–10 minutes to
sterilize the herbs. Strain, and
allow to cool completely.
Store in a sterilized,
airtight, dark glass bottle.
3 To use, pour a little into
a sterilized eyebath and
bathe the eye. If both eyes
are affected, sterilize the
eyebath again and use fresh
mixture to bathe the other eye.

64 EARACHE

Mullein & pasque flower eardrops

Ingredients
*20 drops pasque
flower tincture
24ml infused mullein oil
20 drops goldenseal
tincture*

DOSAGE
Put 2 drops into the ear
3 times a day.

Pasque flower is a good sedative and analgesic that seems to have a specific affinity with the ears, while mullein is a herb with soothing properties that helps repair damaged tissues.

1 Make the tinctures and infused oil (*see Tips 37 and 40*).

2 Combine the ingredients in a sterilized 30ml dropper bottle. Shake.

3 Using the dropper, put 2 drops into the ear and cover with a cotton-wool plug. Leave for 4–6 hours.

PASQUE FLOWER

65 ECZEMA

Heartsease & red clover tea

Ingredients
*20g dried heartsease
20g dried red
clover flowers
20g dried stinging nettle
20g dried burdock
10g dried fumitory
10g dried skullcap
500ml water*

DOSAGE
Take a wineglass dose 3
times a day before meals.

Heartsease is an anti-inflammatory herb and a gentle circulatory stimulant. Like red clover, it also helps clear toxins from the system.

1 Mix the herbs and store in an airtight jar. Spoon 25g of the mixture into a teapot.

2 Pour over freshly boiled water. Infuse for 10 minutes. Strain. Cover and store in a cool place.

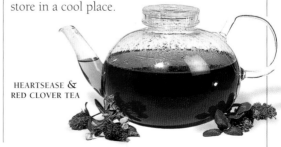

HEARTSEASE & RED CLOVER TEA

66 FACIAL ACNE
Lavender & yarrow facial

Ingredients
5 drops tea tree oil
25ml rosewater
25ml distilled witch hazel
10g dried lavender flowers
10g dried yarrow flowers
10g dried elderflowers
water
DOSAGE
Steam and cleanse
once a day.

In this two-part treatment, steam is used to open the pores and then a lotion is applied to cleanse the skin. The antiseptic and anti-inflammatory herbs that are added to the steam help to combat the symptoms of acne.

1 Combine the tea tree oil with the rosewater and witch hazel to make an astringent lotion.
2 Mix the lavender, yarrow, and elderflowers in a basin and pour boiling water over the mixture.
3 Drape a towel over the head and basin and steam the face for 5–10 minutes, then cleanse with the lotion.

Other treatments
- Eat plenty of fresh fruit and vegetables and take supplements of evening primrose oil, vitamin B-complex, vitamin C, and zinc.
- Blend 3 cabbage leaves with 50ml distilled witch hazel in a food processor and use as a lotion.

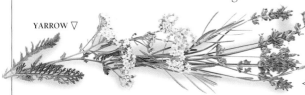

YARROW ▽

◁ LAVENDER

67 COLD SORES

Once infected with the *Herpes simplex* virus, sufferers develop cold sores, usually in the same place, whenever the immune system is under stress. The sores are heralded by a pricking feeling in the skin. Staying fit and healthy is a good preventative. Research has shown that a few herbs display specific antiviral properties and can be used topically to treat infections caused by such viruses. Combine well in a 25ml sterilized dropper bottle the following oils: 8ml tea tree oil, 5ml lavender oil, and 12ml sweet almond oil. To use, dab 1–2 drops of the oil on the affected area every 2 hours.

68 MOUTH ULCERS
Myrrh & rosemary mouthwash

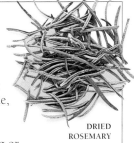

DRIED ROSEMARY

Ingredients
30g dried rosemary
500ml water
15ml myrrh tincture or
5 drops myrrh oil
DOSAGE
Use a wineglass of the
mixture as a mouthwash
every 4 hours until
symptoms ease.

Myrrh is extremely
antimicrobial. However, it
has a fairly unpleasant taste,
so rosemary infusion will
help disguise the flavour.
1 Put the rosemary in a jug or
teapot and add freshly boiled water. Infuse for
10 minutes. Strain.
2 Add the myrrh tincture (*see Tip 37*) or myrrh
oil to the rosemary infusion and stir well. Cover
and store in a cool place.

69 ATHLETE'S FOOT & RINGWORM
Marigold & tea tree ointment

Ingredients
8g beeswax
8g anhydrous lanolin
25ml infused pot marigold
oil
5ml tea tree oil
DOSAGE
Rub gently on affected
areas several times a day
while symptoms persist.

This ointment helps to keep the affected areas
dry, and so discourages fungal growth.
1 Melt the beeswax and anhydrous lanolin in a
double saucepan. Warm the pot marigold oil
(*see Tip 39*) in another double saucepan.
2 Combine the mixtures and remove from the
heat, stirring thoroughly. When the mixture has
started to cool, but before it sets, add the tea
tree oil. Pour into a sterilized dark glass jar and
leave to set.

HERBAL CURE
*Both pot marigold and
tea tree are extremely
antifungal, so are
ideal for treating
athlete's foot.*

△ MARIGOLD & TEA
TREE OINTMENT

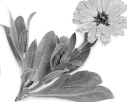

△ POT
MARIGOLD

INFUSED POT △
MARIGOLD OIL

TEA △
TREE OIL

REMEDIES FOR TODDLERS

70 PREVENTATIVE TREATMENTS

Babies have so much to cope with all at once that it is not surprising when occasional health problems arise. However, many minor ailments can be prevented early on by providing a good, balanced diet and a comfortable living environment. Herbs can also be very helpful for babies and toddlers.

> **CAUTION**
> *Consult a doctor if illness persists for more than 2–3 days. For details of dosage, see Tip 42.*

Hyperactivity: Check the diet; avoid synthetic additives and sugar.

Teething: An unavoidable condition, but chamomile or lemon balm infusion eases sore gums.

Sleeplessness: Check the baby is not too hot, cold, hungry, or thirsty.

Rashes & eczema: Rashes may look worse than they really are. Eczema can be related to food allergies.

Colic: Rushed feeding often results in spasms. Slow down feeding time, and drink catmint tea if breastfeeding.

Earache: Often caused by milk allergy, so try soya milk instead of cow's milk.

71 NAPPY RASH

A common affliction, nappy rash can be very painful. Below are several ways to prevent it:
- Check the baby's diet (or the mother's if breastfeeding): the condition can be caused by digestive problems or yeast infections.
- Change nappies frequently, and make sure the baby is well cleaned and dried.
- Use protective, waterproof ointments or infused oils rather than creams.
- Leave the nappy off for as long as possible.
- A good remedy is comfrey and tea tree oil. Make a hot infused oil (*see Tip 40*) using 250g comfrey leaf and 500ml sunflower oil. Add 10ml tea tree oil and mix well. Store in sterilized, dark glass bottles. Apply a little oil to skin that is clean and dry.

COMFREY
This herb increases the rate of cell growth, thereby speeding repair of damaged tissue, while tea tree oil counters infection.

72 CRADLE CAP

Heartsease & marigold oil

HEARTSEASE FLOWERS ▷

Ingredients
100g pot marigold petals
150g heartsease
750ml sunflower oil
DOSAGE
Massage a little of the oil to the affected area several times a day.

Cradle cap is a scaly dermatitis that can affect the scalps of babies. A good herbal remedy is heartsease and marigold oil. Heartsease is a soothing and anti-inflammatory herb, useful for a wide range of skin disorders. Pot marigold is antifungal and astringent, for healing.

1 To make the oil, see Tip 40.

2 Massage oil very gently into the scalp. Be especially careful with newborn babies.

△ HEARTSEASE POWDER

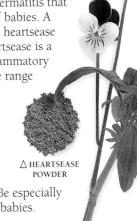

73 COLIC
Catmint tea

Ingredients
10g catmint
175ml water
DOSAGE
Give 25–50ml of the
warm infusion before
meals, reheating
each dose.

Catmint is soothing and ideal for children. It
eases gut spasms and acts as a mild sedative.
1 Place the catmint in a teapot. Add freshly
boiled water and infuse for 10 minutes.
2 Strain and store in a cool place in a
covered jug for up to 48 hours.
Other treatment
▪ If breastfeeding, mothers should
drink an infusion of skullcap,
vervain, wood betony, or
chamomile tea before
feeds (*see Tip 33*).
Check the mother's
and baby's diet for
likely irritants.

CATMINT
TEA

74 SLEEPLESSNESS
Chamomile bath

CHAMOMILE
OIL

Ingredients
2 drops chamomile oil
1 drop lavender oil
DOSAGE
Add the above amounts
of oils to the bath.

Chamomile is one of the best herbs for
small babies – it is sedative and calming,
and an ideal remedy for sleeplessness.
1 Add the oils to the bath.
2 Agitate the water well before
bathing the baby.
Other treatment
▪ Gentle massage can help calm small
babies – stroke arms repeatedly
rather than try an all-over
body massage.
Use 1 drop of
chamomile oil in
20ml of sweet
almond oil.

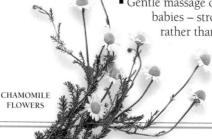
CHAMOMILE
FLOWERS

75 TEETHING
Chamomile & sage gum rub

Ingredients
4 drops chamomile oil
2 drops sage oil
2 drops rosemary oil
20ml sunflower or sweet almond oil
DOSAGE
Rub a small amount on the baby's gums 3–4 times a day.

Chamomile oil acts as a soothing sedative while sage oil is astringent, healing, and antiseptic.

SAGE

1 Pour the oils into a sterilized, dark glass bottle and shake well.
2 Smear a little of the oil on your finger and gently rub it on the baby's gums.
Other treatment
▪ Give 25–50ml of an infusion (*see Tip 33*) of linden flowers or chamomile, before feeds; use 10g dried herb to 500ml water.

76 THREADWORMS IN TODDLERS
Carrot & wormwood mixture

Ingredients
60ml carrot juice
10 drops wormwood tincture
20 drops fennel tincture
DOSAGE
Give a dose each morning before breakfast for 4 days. Repeat 2 weeks later.

CARROT & WORMWOOD MIXTURE

Carrot is toxic for threadworms, and wormwood also clears threadworms from the system. Wormwood has a very bitter taste, so fennel is added to make it more palatable. The mixture below is sufficient for a single dose.
1 Make carrot juice using a food processor or juicer; alternatively, it is available commercially.
2 Stir the tinctures (*see Tip 37*) into the juice.
Other treatment
▪ Finely chop a clove of garlic and mix with a little honey stirred into a cup of warm milk.

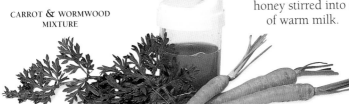

REMEDIES FOR CHILDREN

77 PREVENTATIVE TREATMENTS

On the whole, children's ailments are likely to be mild and self-limiting, and in the developed world, at least, few children face life-threatening disorders. However, children do pick up infections and infestations, and also experience tension and stress. Keeping children healthy, by ensuring they eat well and take plenty of fresh air, can help them fight such attacks. It also helps to limit their reliance on anti-biotics. Herbs are often ideal to treat children's ailments.

Nits: Head lice are common in children. Check the scalp regularly for eggs.

Infections & colds: Repeated use of antibiotics and recurring colds weaken immune systems. Eat well, and take plenty of fresh air.

Upset tummies: Excitement, over-eating, tension, and antibiotics can all lead to stomach upsets.

Bedwetting: Anxiety, infections, and inherited tendencies can result in bedwetting.

Cuts & grazes: These are an inevitable part of childhood. Keep them clean and discourage children from picking the scabs.

REVITALIZING TONIC
American ginseng is an excellent "pick-up" for children who are exhausted or worn down by infections. Give 10 drops of tincture in a little warm water daily.

78 HYPERACTIVITY

Self-heal & wood betony tea

Ingredients

10g dried self-heal spikes
5g dried wood betony
5g dried borage
500ml water

DOSAGE

100–150ml for 3–6 year olds, 3 times a day.

Hyperactive symptoms include sleeplessness, poor attention span, tearfulness, and aggressive behaviour. Food intolerance or pollution are often to blame, or the child may be suffering from emotional difficulties.

Make sure your child's diet contains enough B vitamins, zinc, and iron (found in cereals, meat, and vegetables). Avoid all artificial colourings, preservatives, and additives, and control intake of sugar, milk, and caffeine.

The herbal tea described below will also help hyperactivity: self-heal is cooling and cleansing for the liver, where pollutants and also food additives tend to accumulate. Wood betony has a sedative action on children.

1 Place the dried herbs in a teapot and add freshly boiled water. Infuse for 10 minutes and strain before serving.

2 Flavour with 2–3 drops of liquorice extract/peppermint emulsion per dose. Store in a covered jug in a cool place for up to 48 hours.

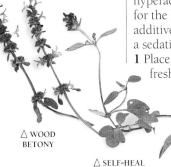

△ WOOD BETONY

△ SELF-HEAL

79 BEDWETTING

Regular bedwetting in young children can be the result of urinary infections, dietary deficiencies, minor physical problems with the urinary tract, or emotional upsets. Seek professional advice to identify the cause of bedwetting in your child.

■ Cornsilk and St John's wort tea is a good remedy for bedwetting. Place 5g dried cornsilk and 10g dried St John's wort in a teapot and add 500ml freshly boiled water. Allow the herb to infuse for 10 minutes and then strain. Give 4-year olds a 100ml dose 3 times a day. Increase the quantity to 150ml for 8-year olds.

80 NITS
Tea tree rinse

TEA TREE ▷

Ingredients
5ml tea tree oil
20 drops lemon oil
500ml water

DOSAGE
Use daily until the
infection clears.

Tea tree oil is extracted
from a tree native to
Australia and is one
of the most
antiseptic and
antibacterial herbs.
Unlike many oils, it does
not irritate the skin. It
is a useful remedy for
nits, the eggs of head lice,
which spread very quickly.
1 Mix the oils in a bottle
and add the warm water.
2 Shake well. Use as a final
rinse after shampooing.

◁ TEA
TREE OIL

81 MUMPS
Thyme & sage gargle

Ingredients
15g dried thyme
15g dried sage
500ml water

DOSAGE
Use every 1–2 hours if
symptoms are severe

In children, mumps is usually mild and suitable
for home treatment. In adolescents and adults,
however, the condition is potentially more
serious, and they should seek professional help.
  Antiseptic gargles and mouthwashes can help
combat the symptoms of mumps. Both thyme
and sage are effective herbs.
1 Place the dried herbs in a teapot and add
freshly boiled water.
2 Infuse for 15 minutes and strain.
3 Use 50ml of the infusion diluted with
50ml of hot water as a gargle. The surplus
may be stored in a covered jug in a
cool place for up to 48
hours.

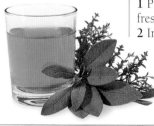

THYME & SAGE
GARGLE

REMEDIES FOR WOMEN

82 PREVENTATIVE TREATMENTS

Each life stage has its distinct strengths or weaknesses and special energy requirements, whether you are young and establishing yourself at work, a mother with young children, or are in the middle or later years. By keeping a good diet and reducing stress, you can alleviate ailments to a large extent. Herbs can help encourage relaxation.

Tension: Stress can cause headaches, so relaxation is vital.

Menopause: Many problems in menopause are helped by herbal tonics, which restore energy to the kidneys.

Gastritis: Too much alcohol and contaminated food are common causes of acute gastritis.

PMS: Taking exercise and avoiding coffee and chocolate can help PMS.

HERBS FOR WOMEN
Certain herbs are particularly good for women's ailments: sage, for example, is known to mimic female hormones, and is therefore a useful supplement during the menopause.

Sprained joints: Sports and exercise can cause joint injuries, which if not remedied in youth can easily lead to arthritis in old age.

83 PREMENSTRUAL SYNDROME

Typical symptoms of premenstrual syndrome (PMS) include emotional upsets, irritability, breast tenderness, food cravings, and digestive irregularities. Symptoms ease when menstruation starts. Relaxation and avoiding stimulants, such as caffeine, can help. There are also several beneficial herbs.

■ Lady's mantle is good for menstrual irregularities, as well as period pain and other gynaecological problems that affect women. Make an infusion (*see Tip 33*) and take one cup 3 times a day. Alternatively, combine 40ml of tincture with 25ml each of black cohosh and black haw tincture, and 10ml of pasque flower tincture. Take 5ml of the mixture 3 times a day. Avoid lady's mantle in pregnancy.

LADY'S MANTLE ▷
Like many herbs with "lady" or "mother" in their name, lady's mantle is a a well-known gynaecological herb.

■ Take 10–20 drops of chaste-tree berry tincture each morning before breakfast (*see Tip 37*).
■ Take 1g daily of evening primrose or borage oils.

84 PERIOD PAIN

One of the best remedies for period cramps is black haw bark – a relaxing herb that has a specific action on the uterus. It works very well when taken on its own, but here it is combined with St John's wort, a restorative nerve tonic, and pasque flower, which has antispasmodic properties.

■ Combine the following tinctures (*see Tip 37*) in a sterilized, dark glass bottle: 15ml black haw bark, 2.5ml St John's wort, 2.5ml pasque flower. Take the whole quantity in a tumbler of warm water when period cramps start. Repeat up to 3 times a day as required.

■ Another remedy is to dilute 10 drops each of cypress, marjoram, and rosemary oil in 20ml of sweet almond oil and gently massage into the abdomen.

85 HEAVY PERIODS
Lady's mantle & shepherd's purse tea

Ingredients
20g dried lady's mantle
10g dried shepherd's purse
10g dried raspberry leaves
*5g dried pot
marigold petals*
5g dried mugwort leaves
500ml water

DOSAGE
Take a teacup dose
3 times a day.

Excessive bleeding is a common menstrual problem. Consult a doctor or herbalist to ensure that no significant causes are involved, and eat plenty of iron-rich foods. This tea will help.
1 Combine the herbs. Place half of the mixture in a teapot or jug. Add the freshly boiled water.
2 Infuse for 10 minutes and strain. Store the surplus in a covered jug in a cool place, and the dry herb mixture in an airtight jar.

LADY'S MANTLE
& SHEPHERD'S
PURSE TEA

86 VAGINAL THRUSH
Marigold & tea tree pessaries

Ingredients
20g cocoa butter
10 drops pot marigold oil
10 drops tea tree oil
5 drops thyme oil

DOSAGE
Insert a pessary into the vagina at night and repeat in the morning while the infection persists.

Pot marigold is a useful antifungal and tea tree is one of the most effective herbal antiseptics available. Thyme oil is antiseptic and antifungal.
1 Melt the cocoa butter in a double boiler or a bowl over hot water.
2 Remove the cocoa butter from the heat and add the oils. Stir well and pour into a pessary mould (available from specialist suppliers).
3 Allow to set (this takes about 4 hours). Remove from the mould. Store in a cool place in an airtight jar or pot lined with greaseproof paper.

THYME

87 VAGINAL ITCHING

At various stages in life, women may experience some vaginal irritation, which can also lead to pain during intercourse. Irritation can be a result of menopausal syndrome, psychological factors, or infection (*see Tip 86*).

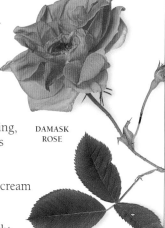

DAMASK ROSE

- An excellent treatment for vaginal itching is damask rose oil, since it is cooling, soothing, astringent, and anti-inflammatory, as well as uplifting. Use 2 drops of rose oil in some distilled witch hazel as a lotion.
- Another remedy is to blend 50g marigold cream with 5 drops of rose oil and as much lady's mantle tincture as can be absorbed by the cream, about 5–10ml. Use morning and night.

88 CYSTITIS (URETHRITIS)

Marshmallow & cornsilk mixture

Ingredients
30ml marshmallow tincture
30ml bearberry tincture
20ml cornsilk tincture
10ml couchgrass tincture
10ml yarrow tincture
DOSAGE
Take 5ml in half a glass of boiling water 4 times a day.

Marshmallow is rich in mucilages to ease inflamed membranes, while yarrow is astringent and healing.
1 Combine the individual tinctures (*see Tip 37*).
2 Store in a sterilized, dark glass bottle. Put 5ml in half a glass of boiling water. Allow to cool, then sip.

Other treatments
- Take 2 x 200mg capsules of echinacea 3 times a day to fight infections.
- Drink plenty of water and avoid alcohol.

CAUTION
Seek professional help if symptoms do not ease after a few days, or if you have fever or loin pain, which may indicate kidney trouble.

89 PRECAUTIONS FOR PREGNANCY

Many herbs should be avoided in pregnancy. Below is a list of some of the herbs to avoid, but always take professional advice. In the first 3 months, avoid all medication.
▪ Do not use the following herbs: arbor vitae, barberry, basil oil, black cohosh, blue cohosh, chamomile oil, *Dang Gui*, feverfew, goldenseal, greater celandine, juniper, lady's mantle, mistletoe, motherwort, mugwort, myrrh, pennyroyal, pokeroot, rue, shepherd's purse, southernwood, tansy, and wormwood.
▪ Do not take alcoholic mixtures during pregnancy.

90 MORNING SICKNESS

Nausea and vomiting are common in pregnancy, beginning in the third or fourth week and lasting up to 3 months. Occasionally they persist throughout pregnancy. Sufferers should consult a doctor if sickness is severe. A few drops of tincture on the tongue can help; try chamomile, ginger, lemon balm, or peppermint.

CRYSTALLIZED GINGER
Ginger is very effective for morning sickness. Take 1g in capsules daily, or chew crystallized ginger.

91 BREASTFEEDING PROBLEMS

Establishing a relaxed pattern of breastfeeding can be difficult for many new mothers. Herbs can help in several ways:
▪ To increase milk flow, make an infusion (*see Tip 33*) of 20g each of fennel seeds and dried nettles, 30g each of dried goat's rue and dried vervain, and 1 tsp powdered cinnamon. Take a cup 4 times a day.
▪ To soothe cracked and sore nipples, apply marigold cream (available over the counter) or a little runny honey mixed with sweet almond oil. Apply frequently.
▪ The breasts may become engorged and painful, and infection (mastitis) may follow. A good remedy is to beat a washed cabbage leaf with a cooking mallet, and place it between the breast and bra.

MARIGOLD CREAM
Apply marigold cream after every feed to soothe cracked or sore nipples.

92 MENOPAUSAL AILMENTS
He Shou Wu & vervain mix

Ingredients
30ml He Shou Wu tincture
20ml vervain tincture
20ml sage tincture
15ml wild yam root tincture
10ml lavender tincture
5ml liquorice tincture

DOSAGE
Take 5ml in a tumbler of warm water 3 times a day before meals.

Menopausal problems in Chinese tradition are associated with run-down kidney energies, so tonics such as *He Shou Wu* that act on the kidney are prescribed. Vervain is a good liver tonic and sedative to calm emotional upsets.

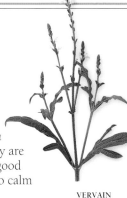

VERVAIN

1 Make the individual tinctures (*see Tip 37*).
2 Mix the tinctures and store in a sterilized, dark glass bottle.

93 IRON-DEFICIENT ANAEMIA
Apricot iron tonic

Ingredients
100ml stinging nettle tincture or juice
50ml dandelion root tincture
250g fresh apricots (wild or organically grown if possible)
500ml water
1 litre red wine
250g honey or sugar

DOSAGE
Take 10ml twice a day.

Apricots are rich in iron and are a good base for this tonic. Stinging nettles and dandelion are added to provide extra nutrients and to stimulate the liver.

1 To make the tinctures, see Tip 37.
2 Put the apricots and water in a pan and bring to the boil. Transfer to a slow cooker and simmer for 12 hours.
3 Allow to cool and remove the stones. Blend in a food processor to produce a fruit pulp.
4 Stir in the tinctures and wine. Store in sterilized, dark glass bottles for 3 months.
Note: Avoid alcoholic mixtures in pregnancy.

APRICOTS

REMEDIES FOR MEN

94 PREVENTATIVE TREATMENTS

A healthy lifestyle when young can prevent many problems from occurring later, while neglect and too much over-indulgence can sow the seeds of long-term ailments in the middle and later years. Whatever your stage of life, keep a healthy diet, exercise, and try to relax, with the help of herbs.

Eyestrain: Have eye-tests regularly: your eyes will become more long-sighted with age.

High blood pressure: *Exercise, weight control, and relaxation will help to reduce blood pressure and risk of heart attacks.*

Prostate problems: *Enlargement of the prostate is common later in life, leading to problems with urination. Seek help without delay.*

Rheumatic aches & pains: Prompt treatment of these as they occur can prevent problems arising later.

Circulatory disorders: Problems of circulation, sometimes manifested as cramp-like pains in the legs, are often associated with smoking.

LATE-ONSET DIABETES
Diabetes may occur late in life, involving excessive thirst, fatigue, and increased urination. It can be hereditary, but can also be caused by decades of a poor diet. Professional help is vital.

95 PROSTATE PROBLEMS
Saw palmetto & Siberian ginseng mix

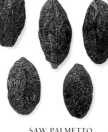

Ingredients
40ml saw palmetto tincture
35ml Siberian ginseng tincture
25ml echinacea tincture
DOSAGE
Take 5ml in half a tumbler of warm water 3 times a day. Increase to 10ml if problem is acute.

Saw palmetto has long been used as a sexual tonic. It is also effective at treating prostate problems, both for inflammation and enlargement. The mix can be used in both cases.

SAW PALMETTO
BERRIES

1 To make the individual tinctures, see Tip 37.
2 Combine the tinctures in a sterilized, dark glass bottle and shake well.

Other treatments
■ Make an infusion (*see Tip 33*) using 10g each of dried white deadnettle, cornsilk, and pellitory-of-the-wall as a healing diuretic tea to help counter prostate enlargement.
■ Take 500mg of evening primrose oil daily.
Note: Do not stop taking long-term medication for prostate problems without medical advice.

CAUTION
If you have a prostate disorder, consult a doctor straight away to eliminate the possibility of prostate cancer.

96 ALOPECIA

While gradual hair loss (baldness) in men occurs with age and is non-reversible, sudden or patchy hair loss (alopecia) can occur in both men and women of any age. It is most common in teenagers and young adults, and may be caused by stress or a vitamin deficiency. The treatments below may be helpful:
■ Apply arnica cream to the bald patches caused by alopecia. Do not use the cream on broken skin, since it can be extremely toxic.

■ Rinse the hair with standard infusions (*see Tip 33*) of rosemary, sage, or stinging nettle.
■ Take vitamin B and evening primrose oil supplements.
■ If stress is likely to be a factor, drink an infusion of equal amounts of skullcap and wood betony (*see Tip 33*).

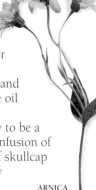

ARNICA

97 IMPOTENCE
Damiana & cinnamon tea

Ingredients
10g dried cinnamon bark
10g Wu Wei Zi (dried schizandra berries)
500ml water
15g dried damiana leaf
DOSAGE
Drink a wineglass dose 3 times a day before meals.

Damiana was used traditionally as an aphrodisiac in South America. Schizandra is used as a sexual tonic for both men and women, enhancing staying power and vigour.
1 Mix the cinnamon, *Wu Wei Zi*, and water in a pan and simmer for 15 minutes to make a decoction.
2 Put the damiana leaf in a teapot and pour on the simmering decoction.
3 Infuse for a further 10 minutes. Strain. Store in a covered jug in a cool place.

DAMIANA

98 HIGH BLOOD PRESSURE
Hawthorn & *Ju Hua* tea

Ingredients
30g dried hawthorn flowering tops
25g Ju Hua (dried, prepared chrysanthemum flowers)
25g dried linden flowers
20g dried yarrow
water
DOSAGE
Drink a teacup dose 3 times a day.

Hawthorn helps to improve the coronary circulation, making the heart more efficient, while chrysanthemum flowers relax the heart and improve blood flow. Maintain regular blood pressure checks.
1 Mix the herbs and store in a dry, airtight jar.
2 Place 2 tsp of the mix in a tisane cup or small teapot. Add a cup of freshly boiled water and infuse for 10 minutes. Strain.

HAWTHORN

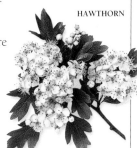

REMEDIES FOR THE ELDERLY

99 PREVENTATIVE TREATMENTS

Old age brings its fair share of health problems as energies wane and the body shows signs of wear and tear. Fatigue, insomnia, and poor appetite are common, and you may experience problems with the digestion, urinary system, and circulation. Stay active, and eat plenty of fresh fruit and vegetables. Vitamin and mineral supplements are very valuable at this time.

Hearing problems: For deafness and tinnitus, try white noise cassette tapes.

Confusion: Short-term memory can become impaired with age. Dried ginkgo leaves and wood betony can help.

Late-onset diabetes: A poor diet can trigger off diabetes later in life (see Tip 94).

Brittle bones: Calcium, magnesium, and exercise help to prevent brittle bones.

Incontinence: Stress incontinence is common in women who have had children and affects both sexes in old age. Horsetail juice can help.

BRITTLE BONES

Sage contains oestrogen-like substances that may help prevent loss of calcium from bones. Take a cup of standard infusion daily (see Tip 33). Alternatively, take a dessertspoon of freshly crushed linseed daily.

100 TONICS FOR THE ELDERLY

Energy levels reduce in old age, and apathy often leads to missed meals. Tonics, as well as food supplements, can therefore be very beneficial in giving the body a little extra boost.

- Take 1–2 x 250mg tablets of American ginseng daily, or a sherry glass of tonic wine.
- Oats are an excellent tonic food, antidepressant, and restorative. Make porridge from freshly milled oatmeal and eat regularly.
- Sage is traditionally associated in the West with longevity. Drink a cup of standard infusion every day (*see Tip 33*).
- Stinging nettles are rich in minerals and vitamins. Drink a cup of infusion daily.
- Cod liver oil reduces the risk of heart disease. Use combined with fish and evening primrose oil capsules (take 500–750mg daily).
- Kelp, or bladderwrack, is rich in iodine and other minerals, and a gentle metabolic stimulant. Take 3–6 x 400mg tablets daily.
- Vitamin B prevents drying at the corners of the mouth and a sore, red tongue. Take 1–2 tablets daily.
- Vitamin C combats infection. Take 1–2g supplement daily.

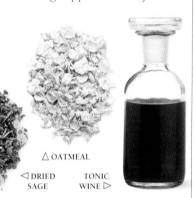

△ OATMEAL

◁ DRIED SAGE   TONIC WINE ▷

101 FORGETFULNESS & CONFUSION

Confusion and forgetfulness are common in old age, and can become senile dementia. This condition needs understanding and patience from the family, as well as professional medical support. There are several herbal remedies that can help to prevent forgetfulness and confusion from occurring:

- Drink a standard infusion of dried ginkgo leaves and wood betony daily (*see Tip 33*). This will improve the circulation to the brain.
- Add 5 drops each of rosemary and basil oils to bathwater as gentle but effective mental stimulants.

GINKGO TABLETS

INDEX

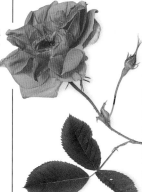

ACKNOWLEDGMENTS

Dorling Kindersley would like to thank:
Hilary Bird for compiling the index;
Marshall Baron for proof reading;
Polly Boyd and Susie Behar for editorial assistance;
and Robert Campbell for DTP assistance.

Photography
KEY: t *top*; b *bottom*; c *centre*; l *left*; r *right*
All photography by Steve Gorton except for:
Mary Evans Picture Library: 9 tr.

Text from this book originally appeared in *Home Herbal*,
published by Dorling Kindersley Ltd. 1995,
and *The Complete Medicinal Herbal*,
published by Dorling Kindersley Ltd. 1993.